CINNAMON, HONEY AND TIGER BONES

Chinese herbal medicine employs many exotic or unexpected substances, as well as the therapeutically powerful ma huang, astragalus and schizandra, to relieve the pain—and remove the cause—of arthritis and related conditions such as gout. Drs. Tsung and Hsu discuss the 40 major herbs and 32 formulas used to treat arthritis, and provide a glossary of scientific terms.

ABOUT THE AUTHORS

Pi-kwang Tsung received his M.S. and Ph.D. from Tokyo University and his M.A. at the University of Kansas. The author of more than 50 scientific papers, Dr. Tsung has served at NYU Medical Center, the University of Connecticut Medical Center, St. Elizabeth's Hospital in Boston and the Dry Eye Institute in Lubbock, Texas. He is President of Technology International, Inc. and Executive Director of the Oriental Healing Arts Institute.

Hong-yen Hsu, who founded the Oriental Healing Arts Institute in 1976, received his doctorate from Meiji University in Tokyo and did research in Japan and in Taiwan, where he taught at several medical colleges and served as director of the Food and Drug Control Bureau of the National Health Administration. He published more than 100 articles and books.

Arthritis and Chinese Herbal Medicine

How ancient, nature-based
treatment has relieved conditions
that afflict tens of millions

Pi-kwang Tsung, Ph.D.
and Hong-yen Hsu, Ph.D.

Keats Publishing, Inc.　　　New Canaan, Connecticut

ARTHRITIS AND CHINESE HERBAL MEDICINE

Copyright © 1987 by Pi-kwang Tsung and Hong-yen Hsu

ISBN: 0-87983-735-7

Printed in the United States of America

Good Health Guides are published by
Keats Publishing, Inc.
27 Pine Street (Box 876)
New Canaan, Connecticut 06840-0876

Contents

Arthritis and Chinese Herbal Medicine

We frequently receive desperate phone calls and letters from arthritis victims who complain about the side effects of Western medicines and want us to recommend a Chinese medicine to ease their pain, since we have published many books on Chinese herbal therapy. For example, one correspondent wrote: "According to Western medicine the medicine for arthritis is aspirin. Unfortunately my stomach cannot tolerate aspirin any more. In September 1984, I had major surgery and half of my stomach was cut away. I am looking for the right medicine for my arthritis and would like to have your honest opinion."

Arthritis causes more prolonged pain to more Americans than any other disease. At least seven million Americans are reported to be afflicted with constant arthritis pain. Although more than 33 million dollars have been spent on arthritis-related research through the National Institutes of Health, an estimated 70 million work-days were lost because of arthritis during the past year; some 500,000 sufferers required hospitalization. The personal tragedies that this involves can only be guessed at from the letters we have received from arthritis victims.

In rheumatoid arthritis, researchers believe that the

body's immune system is not working properly. Gout, another form of arthritis, is a disease of metabolic disorder. Arthritis can be called a patient-specific syndrome. Every biologically unique arthritis patient has his or her own body chemistry and immune system which determines his or her particular immune response.

The principle of Chinese medicine is to diagnose symptoms or illnesses in terms of the patient's individuality. Most Chinese herbal formulas are designed not only to relieve symptomatic pain but more importantly to enhance the body's immune system by stimulating metabolism and the function of the endocrine system. Therefore, Chinese medicine, as a patient-specific therapy, is well suited to the treatment of arthritis, a patient-specific syndrome. The Japanese are already treating arthritis patients with Chinese herbal formulas with remarkable success.

This small book is an endeavor to help American physicians and patients to understand the use of Chinese herbal therapy in the management of arthritis.

WHAT IS RHEUMATOID ARTHRITIS?

Rheumatoid arthritis is an inflammatory disease of connective tissue with major symptoms in joint swelling and pain. The initial stage of rheumatoid arthritis is marked by symmetrical swelling and pain in the joints of the fingers, hands, and knees. Gradually the joints are destroyed and deformed, so that they are less and less able to function. Eventually the joints become immobile.

It has been suggested that a pathogen-like virus causes the disease. However, there is no strong evidence to support this theory. The theory that it is an autoimmune disorder is supported by two observations: (i) the C-reactive protein in the immunoglobulin fraction is increased in the serum of rheumatoid arthritis patients, and (ii) denatured immunoglobulin (IgG), called "the Rheumatoid factor," is increased in the serum of these patients. Therefore, it seems likely that complexes of IgG and anti-IgG antibodies are deposited in the joints, their presence eliciting the inflammatory reactions leading to swelling and pain in the joints (see Fig. 1).

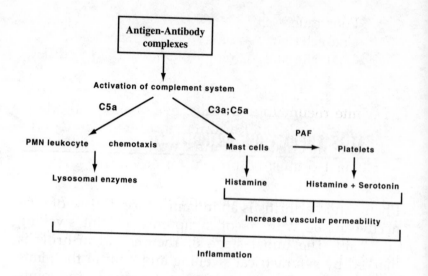

FIGURE 1
Pathways to inflammation triggered by antigen-antibody complexes.
PAF=platelet activating factor
PMN=polymorphonuclear

Diagnostic Criteria

The American Rheumatism Association has approved a set of criteria for the diagnosis of rheumatoid arthritis. The eleven components of the criteria are as follows:
(1) Morning stiffness
(2) Pain on motion of one joint
(3) Swelling of one joint
(4) Swelling of at least one other joint
(5) Symmetrical joint swelling
(6) Subcutaneous nodules
(7) Typical x-ray change
(8) Positive rheumatoid factor test

(9) Poor mucin clot
(10) Characteristic histology of synovial biopsy
(11) Characteristic histology of rheumatoid nodule

Classical rheumatoid arthritis: seven or more criteria
Definite rheumatoid arthritis: five or more criteria
Probable rheumatoid arthritis: three or more criteria
Possible rheumatoid arthritis: two or more criteria
Criteria 1–5 must be present for at least 6 weeks.

These criteria allow for comparative studies of patients by different physicians in different communities. At the individual physician/patient level, the criteria are often of little use in early manifestations of the disease.

WESTERN MEDICINE AND RHEUMATOID ARTHRITIS

There is no drug that can cure chronic rheumatoid arthritis at the present time. The drugs used for its treatment merely control the symptoms and ease pain by suppressing or masking symptoms. Those most commonly used are steroids, non-steroid anti-inflammatory drugs, anti-rheumatoid agents and immunosuppressors or immunomodulators.

Steroids

Steroids are the most commonly used drugs for arthritis. However, they cannot cure arthritis; they can only ease the pain by suppressing the symptoms. The principal complications resulting from prolonged therapy with steroids are fluid and electrolyte disturbances; hyperglycemia and glycosuria; susceptibility to infections, including tuberculosis; peptic ulcer, which may bleed or perforate; osteoporosis; a characteristic myopathy; psychosis; and Cushing's syndrome, consisting of "moon face," "buffalo hump," supraclavicular fat pads, "central obesity," striae, ecchymoses, acne, and hirsutism.

Nonsteroid anti-inflammatory drugs

The most common nonsteroid anti-inflammatory drugs are aspirin, phenylbutazone, and indomethacin. These drugs are for short-term usage only. Long-term use of these drugs can result in such complications as gastric ulceration and bleeding, abdominal pain, skin eruption, CNS disturbances, and disturbance in the acid-base balance and electrolyte structure of blood plasma.

Antirheumatoid agents

Gold compounds and penicillamine are commonly used antirheumatoid agents. These agents are anti-inflammatory, but they have no direct effect upon pain. Although they appear to induce a remission in active rheumatoid arthritis, the drawback of these agents is their potential for damage to the kidneys and blood, requiring periodic urine and blood tests.

Immunosuppressors and immunomodulators

Anticancer drugs which have an immunosuppressive effect have been applied (i.e. cyclophosphamide, 6-methylpurine, azathioprine). The usual side effects of immunosuppressors are anorexia, nausea, and vomiting; long-term use may increase the incidence of some cancers, infections and bone marrow suppression.

These very dangerous immunosuppressive drugs suppress the body's immune system and the body needs its immune system's protective powers to defend against other illness.

All of these drugs have been used for treating rheumatoid arthritis by combining the four different types according to patients' symptoms. However, there is no fundamental formula for treatment.

In addition to drug therapy, physical, diet, acupuncture, and surgical therapies have been used.

CHINESE HERBAL FORMULAS AND RHEUMATOID ARTHRITIS

In Chinese medicine the term "moisture disease" has no Western medical equivalent, but it has been generally translated as "wind and moisture disease," a phrase which is now commonly used. One of the first references to "wind and moisture disease" appears in *Chin kuei yao lueh,* where it is used to define an illness accompanied by generalized pain.

Chinese medical theory holds that diseases are brought about by either internal or external causes. External causes arise mainly from geography, weather, and environment and are known as the "six excesses": wind, dryness, cold, fire, moisture, and heat. Because "wind and moisture fight each other," the patient feels severe bone and joint pain, making it very difficult for him to stretch or bend. As early as *Huang ti nei ching,* "wind and moisture" was described as one of the "numb diseases" in Chinese medicine. A "numb disease" is characterized by an increase of pain due to cold or damp weather.

Formulas for Rheumatic Fever and Early-Stage Rheumatoid Arthritis

Rheumatic fever usually starts with an acute inflammation and painful swelling of the joints; before the condition is brought under control, many of its victims are left with permanently damaged hearts. While most cases start with painful swelling in the joints, it is well to remember that the acute inflammatory process does not always limit itself to the joints. The heart, the blood vessels, the kidneys, the nerves, and other organs of the body are often involved, while occasionally the joints themselves are free and clear.

For rheumatic fever and the early stage of rheumatoid arthritis *Ma-huang-chia-chu-tang* and *Ma-hsing-i-kan-tang* are commonly used formulas (see Table 1).

TABLE 1.
Components of *Ma-huang-chia-chu-tang* and *Ma-hsing-i-kan-tang*

Ma-huang-chia-chu-tang	Ma-hsing-i-kan-tang
Ma-huang	Ma-huang
Apricot seed	Apricot seed
Licorice	Licorice
Cinnamon	Coix
Gypsum	
Atractylodes (white)	

Ma-huang, apricot seed, and licorice are the common components in the two formulas.

Ma-huang contains the chemical compounds ephedrine, pseudoephedrine (Fig. 2), N-methylephedrine, and N-methylpseudoephedrine as its major active components. These chemical compounds have been shown to have anti-inflammatory activity.

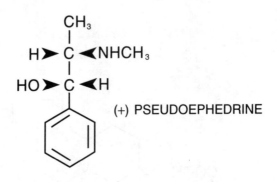

FIGURE 2
One of the anti-inflammatory components of Ma-huang

Apricot seed is considered to be an excellent health food for the throat, and is commonly used as cough medicine and in the treatment of bronchial asthma. It is also considered to have a mucoregulator function. Vocalists frequently use a drink made from apricot seed to maintain the quality and strength of their voices. Amygdalin[17], ß-glucosidase[1,8,13], amino-pepitdase[14], and steroid compounds estrone and estradiol-ß-17-ol[4] have been identified in the apricot seed. However, the pharmacologically active components are not necessarily limited to these materials.

Licorice contains glycyrrhizin (Fig. 3), which is known to have anti-inflammatory activity and stimulatory activity in reticuloendothelial systems.[12,20]

Cinnamon possesses antibacterial properties[16], and atractylodes contain anti-histamine compounds ß-eudesmol and hinesol.[6] An infusion of coix is considered nutritive, refrigerant, and diuretic; alcohol fermented from the seeds is considered antirheumatic. Coixol isolated from coix has a muscle-relaxing effect.

Ma-hsing-i-kan-tang and *Ma-huang-chia-chu-tang* are also effective in other forms of arthritis.

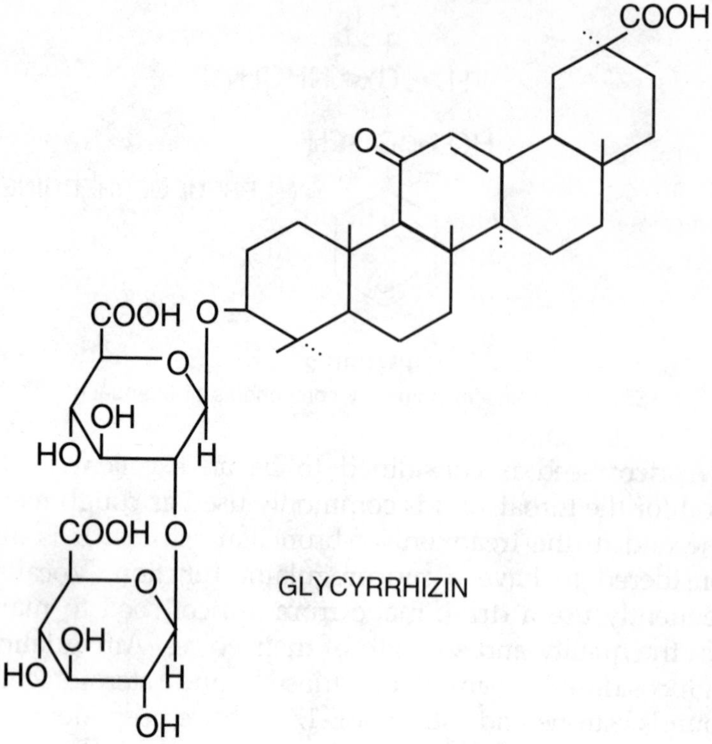

GLYCYRRHIZIN

FIGURE 3

Chinese Herbal Medicines and Chronic Rheumatoid Arthritis

Because of the hazardous side effects of Western medications, Chinese herbal medicine has become increasingly popular in Japan, Taiwan, and Mainland China for the treatment of chronic rheumatoid arthritis.

Kuei-chih-chia-ling-chu-fu-tang is the most widely prescribed Chinese herbal medicine in Japan. In cases of rheumatic fever and early-stage rheumatoid arthritis, the prescribed Chinese herbal formulas contain ma-huang as the anti-inflammatory component. However, aconite is the key component in the herbal formulas for chronic rheumatoid arthritis. Aconite content in the formulas is increased according to the stage of the disease; a smaller amount is prescribed for acute rheumatoid arthritis.

Aconite contains aconitine ($C_{34}H_{47}NO_{11}$) and related alkaloids. The fresh herb is extremely toxic, but in the dried root much of the aconitine has decomposed to picroaconitine and aconine, which are less toxic.[11]

Aconite was prescribed in twenty of the formulas listed in *Shang han lun,* and in 29 of the formulas in *Chin kuei yao lueh.* Its popularity is due to the stimulatory effect that it has on metabolism and its ability to control pain.

Aconite is used not only in *Kuei-chih-chia-ling-chu-*

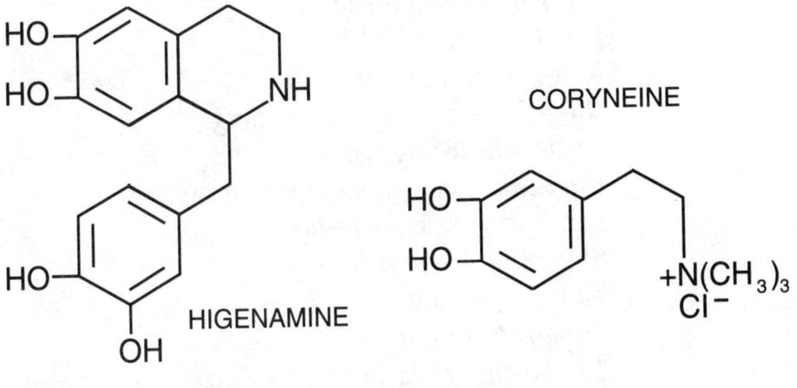

FIGURE 4
Structures of higenamine and coryneine

fu-tang, *Kan-tsao-fu-tzu-tang* and other formulas for rheumatoid arthritis, neuralgia, and hemiplegia, but also in *Pa-wei-ti-huang-wan* and other herbal formulas for diseases of old age, e.g. diabetes, lower back pain, and skin disease, and in *Chen-wu-tang* for chronic diarrhea.

Cardiotonic effect is also found in aconite. In addition to aconitine and related alkaloids, a cardiotonic compound higenamine[10] and a hypertensive compound coryneine[9] have been isolated from aconite (see Fig. 4).

The Chinese herbal formulas commonly used in Japan for chronic rheumatoid arthritis are as follows[19]:

> *Chai-hu-kuei-chih-tang*
> *Chai-hu-kuei-chih-kan-chiang-tang*
> *Fang-chi-huang-chi-tang-chia-fu-tzu*
> *Hsia-yu-hsieh-tang*
> *Hsiao-chai-hu-tang*
> *Huang-lien-chieh-tu-tang*
> *I-yi-jen-tang*
> *I-yi-jen-tang-chia-pao-fu-tzu*
> *Jen-shen-tang*
> *Kan-tsao-fu-tzu-tang*
> *Kuei-chih-chia-ling-chu-fu-tang*
> *Kuei-chih-fu-ling-wan*
> *Kuei-chih-shao-yao-chih-mu-tang*
> *San-huang-hsieh-hsin-tang*
> *Shu-ching-huo-hsieh-tang*
> *Ta-chai-hu-tang*
> *Ta-fang-feng-tang*
> *Tao-ho-cheng-chi-tang*
> *Ti-tang-tang*
> *Yueh-pi-chia-chu-tang*

Kenpo-gan

The Chinese herbal medicine *Kenpo-gan* has become very popular among rheumatoid arthritis patients in Japan. *Kenpo-gan* originated in Taiwan and Mainland China under the name *Pai-hsien-pi-chien-pu-wan*.

Kenpo-gan contains the following ingredients:

Achyranthes
Astragalus
Atractylodes (red)
Atractylodes (white)
Chiang-huo
Cuscuta
Dioscorea
Eucommia
Ginseng
Honey
Lycium
Peony
Phellodendron
Psoralea
Rehmannia
Schizandra
Siler
Sinomenium
Tang-kuei
Tiger bone
Tortoise shell

Kenpo-gan is approved by the Japanese Food and Drug Administration as a Chinese herbal medicine and is widely used in clinics for the treatment of rheumatoid arthritis in Japan. Among 103 patients tested in one study, 41 patients showed striking improvement, with some effectiveness in another 47 patients. Only 13 patients did not respond to the formula.[18] Thus more than 86 percent of these patients derived some benefit from taking *Kenpo-gan*.

EFFICACY OF STEROID DRUGS WITH CHINESE HERBAL FORMULAS

The combination of steroid drugs and Chinese herbal medicines has also been demonstrated in numerous clinical trials to enhance the efficacy of steroid drugs used in the treatment of allergies. Although the disadvantages of the potential side effects are obvious, the advantage of steroids in easing pain quickly and for a relatively long period is not to be denied. Fortunately, when certain Chinese herbal formulas are combined with steroids they have been found to minimize the risk of such side effects.[2,3,7,18]

GOUT

In Western medicine gout is classified as a joint disease which is characterized by acute arthritic pain in the peripheral joints: the disease is caused by abnormal metabolism of uric acid. In over 95 percent of the cases, the excessive serum urate concentration results in hyperuricemia. The arthritic pain of gout is due to the deposit of uric acid crystals around the joint. Urate deposits may also appear in other parts of the body as tophi. The deposit of monosodium urate crystals in the kidneys, however, may result in serious kidney damage. Excess excretion of uric acid through the kidneys may produce kidney stones (10%–20% of the cases), while deficient excretion may result in hyperuricemia.

Gout often affects those who eat and drink excessively. Most patients are over 40 years old, and about seventy percent are obese. The ratio of male to female patients is 20:1.

There are two types: acute gouty arthritis and chronic gout. The onset of the disease is frequently sudden. The first attack usually occurs at the metatarsophalangeal joint of the great toe, though it may also occur at finger, wrist, ankle, or knee joints. Two to three hours after the pain begins, the joint becomes swollen and excruciatingly tender, and the skin turns dark red. Although the joint function returns to normal after the first attack, such episodes may recur after several months or even two years. As the disease progresses, the attacks become more frequent and more severe. Without prophylactic therapy, chronic gout may develop.

The usual therapy for patients with gout is colchicine, a drug derived from the autumn crocus and discovered in ancient Egypt. Since a side effect of colchicine may be acute diarrhea, the drug should be taken only as directed by a physician.

Other drugs which are frequently prescribed for gout are Benemid and Anturan, both of which increase the excretion of uric acid and thereby promptly lower the plasma uric acid level. The side effects are stimulation of the central nervous system, gastrointestinal irritation, convulsions, and possible death from respiratory failure.

Chinese Medicine and Gout

In *Shang han lun* and *Chin kuei yao lueh* there is no mention of any term for gout. Since foods were prepared in a simple manner in ancient China, perhaps the disease did not exist. However, during the Yuan Dynasty, the term for gout appeared in *Ko chih yu lun*.

In Chinese medicine, the word for gout means "painful numbness" or "numb pain." According to the medical classics, other terms for gout include "evil wind," "numb disease," "seasonal disease," or "white tiger pain" (since the pain is sharp like a tiger's bite). The symptoms of the disease are acute pain in various joints throughout the body, weakness of both ch'i and blood, and immobility of the joints. If the pain is very acute, the disease is called "white tiger seasonal disease." The use of the various terms for gout in Chinese medicine closely parallels the definitions in modern Western medicine. The so-called "gout of old age" probably refers to gouty arthritis or rheumatism.

According to the principles of Chinese medicine, gout occurs when the "seven sentiments" are attacked by chills, moisture, and wind. The objectives of therapy are regulation of the circulation of ch'i and blood in the blood vessels and relief of the patient's nervous tension.

The most popular formula prescribed by modern Chinese physicians for treating gout is *Tang-kuei-lien-tung-tang*. This formula serves as an anodyne.

Clinical Treatment of Gout in Japan

For treating acute pain during attacks of gout, Dr. K. Okano[15] uses *Wu-tou-tang, Kuei-chih-chia-ling-chu-fu-tang,* and *Kan-tsao-fu-tzu-tang* to relieve the pain. These formulas function as diuretics and analgesics.

Before and after each attack of gout, Dr. Okano prescribes *Yueh-pi-chia-chu-tang* for strong-conformation patients, and *Fang-chi-huang-chi-tang* with either *Ma-huang-tang* or *Yueh-pi-chia-chu-tang* for weak-conformation patients.

During the periods between attacks, *Ta-chai-hu-tang* and bupleurum derivatives are given.

Japanese references list the following Chinese formulas for treating and preventing gout:

Fang-chi-huang-chi-tang: This formula is recommended for obese patients with weakness of the muscles.

Fang-feng-tung-sheng-san: This formula is suitable for obese patients.

Kuei-chih-chia-ling-chu-fu-tang or *Kuei-chih-erh-yueh-pi-i-chia-chu-fu-tang.*

Ta-chai-hu-tang: This formula is suitable for patients having abdominal distention with pain and resistance.

Wu-tou-tang: This formula is an anodyne during attacks of gout, and helps to alleviate the accompanying symptoms.

CONCLUDING REMARKS

The value of Chinese herbal medicine in the treatment of arthritis can be summarized as follows:

(1) Western medicines used for the treatment of arthritis include steroids, nonsteroid anti-inflammatory drugs, antirheumatoid agents and immunosuppressors or immunomodulators. These drugs can only control the symptoms and ease the pain of arthritis. However, the incidence of hazardous side effects with these drugs is high. In the course of more than 2,000 years of clinical experience with billions of people, a number of Chinese herbal formulas have been developed for the effective treatment of arthritis. The identification of many of their active chemical components during the past fifty years has made it more easy for us to understand how Chinese herbs act upon arthritis.

(2) Many Chinese herbal formulas have been approved for use in physicians' prescriptions in Japan, and are covered by Japanese National Health Insurance.

(3) The combination of Chinese herbal medicines and steroid drugs can reduce the amount of steroid to be used by enhancing the steroid effect, which is very beneficial to patients since it can minimize side effects.

(4) We think that it is important that both the public in general and American physicians in particular become aware of the role that Chinese herbal formulas can play in the treatment of arthritis. It is partly for this reason that we have introduced the active chemical compounds isolated from Chinese herbs wherever this evidence is relevant.

(5) We hope that this small book will encourage more American physicians to consider the use of Chinese herbal formulas in treating their arthritis patients.

GLOSSARY OF TERMS

Alkaloid
One of a large group of organic basic substances found in plants. Examples are atropine, caffeine, morphine, nicotine, quinine.

Antibody
An immunoglobulin molecule that interacts only with the antigen that induced its synthesis in lymphoid tissue.

Antigen
Any substance which is capable of inducing the formation of antibodies and of reacting specifically in some detectable manner with the antibodies so induced.

Ch'i (氣)
"Vital essence." This would correspond to the life force, or stock of vitality which must be maintained to ensure health. The idea of ch'i is fundamental to Chinese medical thinking, and no one English word or phrase can adequately capture its meaning.

Complement
The nonspecific factor in fresh serum needed to bring about lysis of a foreign invader. The complement

system consists of an elaborate set of interacting proteins.

Diuretic
(1) increasing the secretion of urine
(2) an agent that promotes the secretion of urine

Immunoglobulin
A protein of animal origin endowed with known antibody activity.

Immunomodulator
An agent which can adjust and/or regulate immune responsiveness.

Immunosuppressor
An agent which can check or reduce the severity of immune responsiveness.

Lysosome
One of the minute bodies seen with the electron microscope in many types of cells, containing various hydrolytic enzymes and normally involved in the process of localized intracellular digestion.

Mast Cell
A blood cell which releases histamine upon antigen-mediated or antibody-mediated degranulation.

Mucoregulator
An agent which controls mucus secretion.

Neutrophil
A blood cell. A granular leukocyte having a nucleus with three to five lobes connected by slender threads of chromatin, and cytoplasm containing five inconspicuous granules; called also polymorphonuclear (PMN) leukocyte.

Platelet
A disk-shaped structure found in the blood of all mammals and chiefly known for its role in blood coagulation.

Tophi
Plural of tophus. A chalky deposit of urate found in the tissues about the joints in gout.

GLOSSARY OF HERBS

Achyranthes (root)
Achyranthes bidentata, niu-hsi (牛膝)
Aconite
Aconitum carmichaeli, A. Kusnezoffii, fu-tzu (附子)
Alisma (root)
Alisma plantago-aquatica, A. orientale, tse-hsieh (澤瀉)
Anemarrhena
Anemarrhena asphodeloides, chih-mu (知母)
Apricot (seed)
Prunus armeniaca, hsing-jen (杏仁)
Astragalus (root)
Astragalus hoantchy, A. chinensis, huang-chi (黄耆)
Atractylodes (red rhizome)
Atractylodes lancea, A. chinensis, A. japonica, tsang-shu
(蒼术)
Atractylodes (white rhizome)
Atractylodes macrocephala, A. lancea, pai-shu (白术)
Capillaris
Artemisia capillaris, yin-chen-hao (茵陳蒿)
Chiang-huo (rhizome)
Notopterygium spp., *chiang-huo* (羌活)
Cimicifuga
Cimicifuga dahurica, C. foetida, C. heracleifolia, sheng-ma (升麻)

Cinnamon (twigs)
Cinnamomum cassia, kuei-chih (桂枝)
Coix (seed)
Coix lachryma-jobi, i-yi-jen (薏苡仁)
Cuscuta (seed)
Cuscuta chinensis, C. japonica, tu-szu (菟絲子)
Dioscorea (rhizome)
Dioscorea batatis, D. opposita, shan-yao (山藥)
Eucommia (bark)
Eucommia ulmoides, tu-chung (杜仲)
Ginger (raw rhizome)
Zingiber officinale, sheng-chiang (生薑)
Ginseng (raw root)
Panax ginseng, jen-shen (人參)
Ginseng (steamed root)
Panax ginseng, hung-shen (紅參)
Gypsum
Calcium sulfate ($CaSO_42H_2O$), *shih-kao* (石膏)
Honey
Mel (Apis chinensis, A. cerana), feng-mi (蜂密)
Jujube (fruit)
Zizyphus sativa, Z. vulgaris, ta-tsao (大棗)
Licorice (root)
Glycyrrhiza uralensis, G. glabra var. *glandulifera, kan-tsao* (甘草)
Lycium (fruit)
Lycium chinensis, kou-chi-tzu (枸杞子)
Ma-huang
Ephedra sinica, E. equisetina, ma-huang (麻黃)
Peony (white root)
Paeonia lactiflora, shao-yao (芍藥)
Phellodendron (bark)
Phellodendron amurense, huang-pai (黃柏)

Polyporus
Polyporus grifona umbellata, P. umbellatus, chu-ling (豬苓)

Psoralea (seed)
Psoralea corylifolia, pu-ku-chih (補骨脂)

Pueraria (root)
Pueraria thunbergiana, ko-ken (葛根)

Rehmannia (steam-dried root)
Rehmannia glutinosa, shu-ti-huang (熟地黃)

Schizandra (fruit)
Schizandra chinensis, wu-wei-tzu (五味子)

Scute (root)
Scutellaria baicalensis, huang-chin (黃芩)

Siler (root)
Ledebouriella seseloides, L. saposhnikovia divaricata, Siler divaricatum, fang-feng (防風)

Sinomenium (stem and rhizome)
Sinomenium acutum, han-fang-chi (漢防己)

Sophora (root)
Sophora subprostrata, tou-ken (山豆根)

Tang-kuei (root)
Angelica sinensis, A. acutiloba, tang-kuei (當歸)

Tiger bone
Os Tigris [Panthera tigris], hu-ku (虎骨)

Tortoise shell
Carapax Amydae [Amyda sinensis], pieh-chia (鱉甲)

GLOSSARY OF FORMULAS

Chai-hu-kuei-chih-tang (柴胡桂枝湯)
Bupleurum and Cinnamon Combination
Chai-hu-kuei-chih-kan-chiang-tang (柴胡桂枝乾薑湯)
Bupleurum, Cinnamon, and Ginger Combination
Chen-wu-tang (真武湯)
Vitality Combination
Fang-chi-huang-chi-tang (防己黃耆湯)
Stephania and Astragalus Combination
Fang-chi-huang-chi-tang-chia-fu-tzu
(防己黃耆湯加附子)
Stephania and Astragalus Combination with Aconite
Fang-feng-tung-sheng-san (防風過聖散)
Siler and Platycodon Formula
Hsia-yu-hsieh-tang (下瘀血湯)
Persica and Eupolyphaga Combination
Hsiao-chai-hu-tang (小柴胡湯)
Minor Bupleurum Combination
Huang-lien-chieh-tu-tang (黃連解毒湯)
Coptis and Scute Combination
I-yi-jen-tang (薏苡仁湯)
Coix Combination
I-yi-jen-tang-chia-pao-fu-tzu (薏苡仁湯加炮附子)
Coix Combination with Processed Aconite

Jen-shen-tang (人參湯)
Ginseng Combination

Kan-tsao-fu-tzu-tang (甘草附子湯)
Licorice and Aconite Combination

Kenpo-gan (健步丸)
Health-Promoting Formula (*Pai-hsien-pi-chien-pu-wan*)

Kuei-chih-chia-ling-chu-fu-tang (桂枝加苓术附湯)
Cinnamon and Atractylodes Combination

Kuei-chih-erh-yueh-pi-i-chia-chu-fu-tang
(桂枝二越婢－加术附湯)
Cinnamon, Ma-huang, and Gypsum Combination
with Atractylodes and Hoelen

Kuei-chih-fu-ling-wan (桂枝茯苓丸)
Cinnamon and Hoelen Combination

Kuei-chih-shao-yao-chih-mu-tang (桂枝芍藥知母湯)
Cinnamon and Anemarrhena Combination

Ma-hsing-i-kan-tang (麻杏薏甘湯)
Ma-huang and Coix Combination

Ma-huang-tang (麻黃湯)
Ma-huang Combination

Ma-huang-chia-chu-tang (麻黃加术湯)
Ma-huang and Atractylodes Combination

Pa-wei-ti-huang-wan (八味地黃丸)
Rehmannia Eight Formula

Pai-hsien-pi-chien-pu-wan (百仙碑健步丸)
Health-Promoting Formula (=*Kenpo-gan*)

San-huang-hsieh-hsin-tang (三黃瀉心湯)
Coptis and Rhubarb Combination

Shu-ching-huo-hsieh-tang (疎經活血湯)
Clematis and Stephania Combination

Ta-chai-hu-tang (大柴胡湯)
Major Bupleurum Combination

Ta-fang-feng-tang (大防風湯)
Major Siler Combination

Tang-kuei-lien-tung-tang（當歸拈痛湯）
Tang-kuei and Anemarrhena Combination
Tao-ho-cheng-chi-tang（桃核承氣湯）
Persica and Rhubarb Combination
Ti-tang-tang（抵當湯）
Rhubarb and Leech Combination
Wu-tou-tang（烏頭湯）
Wu-tou Combination
Yueh-pi-chia-chu-tang（越婢加朮湯）
Atractylodes Combination

HERBAL FORMULAS RECOMMENDED FOR RHEUMATOID ARTHRITIS AND GOUT

Rheumatoid Arthritis

early stage: *I-yi-jen-tang, Ma-hsing-i-kan-tang*
late stage *(chronic): Kuei-chih-chia-ling-chu-fu-tang*
for pain: *tang-kuei-lien-tung-tang*

Gout

Tang-kuei-lien-tung-tang

I-yi-jen-tang:
Ma-huang...........4.0	Tang-kuei 4.0	Coix............8.0
Atractylodes	Cinnamon 3.0	Peony........3.0
(red) 4.0		
Licorice 2.0		

Ma-hsing-i-kan-tang:
Ma-huang...........4.0	Apricot seed 3.0
Licorice 2.0	Coix...................10.0

Kuei-chih-chia-ling-chu-fu-tang:
Cinnamon 4.0	Peony..................3.0	Jujube........3.0
Ginger (raw)......3.0	Licorice...............1.5	Hoelen......5.0
Atractylodes	Aconite 0.5–1.0	
(red) 5.0		

Tang-kuei-lien-tung-tang:

Tang-kuei	2.5	Anemarrhena	2.5	Chiang-huo	2.5
Capillaris	2.5	Atractylodes (red)	2.0	Scute	2.5
Polyporus	2.5	Alisma	2.5	Siler	2.0
Pueraria	2.0	Ginseng (raw)	2.0	Sophora	1.0
Atractylodes (white)	2.5	Cimicifuga	1.0		
Licorice	1.0				

Note: The unit of dosages is given in grams, and the dosage indicated for each formula is the maximum daily amount allowed. If there are no directions for administration given after a formula, the formula is decocted in the conventional way, that is, a one-day dosage of the formula is added to 500 ml of water and decocted until 300 ml remains; then the dregs are discarded and the decoction is divided into two or three portions. Each portion is taken warmed one hour before meals, or on an empty stomach. Dosages may vary according to the patient's size and strength, and the severity of the disease.

SUGGESTED READINGS

Hsu, Hong-yen and Peacher, William G. **Chinese Herb Medicine and Therapy.** New Canaan, Conn.: Keats Publishing/OHAI, 1994.

Hsu, Hong-yen and Peacher, William G. **Chen's History of Chinese Medical Science.** Los Angeles: Oriental Healing Arts Institute, 1977.

Hsu, Hong-yen. **How to Treat Yourself with Chinese Herbs.** New Cannan, Conn.: Keats Publishing/OHAI, 1994.

Tsung, Pi-kwang and Hsu, Hong-yen. **Immunology and Chinese Herbal Medicine.** Long Beach, CA: Oriental Healing Arts Institute, 1986.

Tsung, Pi-kwang and Hsu, Hong-yen. **Allergy and Chinese Herbal Medicine.** Long Beach, CA: Oriental Healing Arts Institute, 1977.

Bulletin of the Oriental Healing Arts Institute (1976–1985)/**Oriental Healing Arts International Bulletin** (1986–). Dr. Hong-yen Hsu, editor 1976–1986. Dr. Pi-Kwang Tsung, editor 1987.

CLASSICAL REFERENCES

Chang, Chung-ching. **Chin kuei yao lueh** (Prescriptions from the Golden Chamber). Han dynasty (219 A.D.). [English translation by Hsu, Hong-yen and Wang, Su-yen (Long Beach, CA.; Oriental Healing Arts Institute, 1983).]

Shang han lun (Treatise on Febrile Diseases). Han dynasty (219 A.D.). [English translation by Hsu, Hong-yen and Peacher, William G. (Los Angeles: Oriental Healing Arts Institute, 1981).]

Chu, Tan-hsi (aka Chu, Cheng-heng). **Ko chih yu lun** (Principles of Diagnosis and Treatment). Yuan dynasty (1347 A.D.).

Wang, Ping. **Huang ti nei ching** (The Yellow Emperor's Treatise on Internal Medicine). Tang dynasty (762 A.D.) [English translation by Lu, Henry C. (Vancouver, B.C.; Academy of Oriental Heritage, 1978).]

REFERENCES

1. Akabori, A. and Kagawa, S. *Shoyakugaku Zasshi* (Japanese Journal of Pharmacognosy) 37(1983): 241.
2. Arichi, S. *Iyaku to Yakugaku* (Medical and Pharmaceutical Science) 8(1982) no. 2: 415.
3. ——— and Kotani, T. *Iyaku* (Medicine) 16(1980): 1285.
4. Awad, O. *Phytochemistry* 13(1974): 678.
5. Hikino, H. et al. *Chemical and Pharmaceutical Bulletin* 28(1980): 2900.
6. Itokawa, H. et al. *Tennen Yakubutsu no Kaihatsu to Oyo Shinpojumu Koenyoshishu* (Abstracts of the Proceedings of the Symposium on the Development and Application of Natural Products) 3(1980): 4.
7. Kaneko, M. *Gendai Toyo Igaku* (Journal of Traditional Sino-Japanese Medicine) 2(1981) no. 3: 28.
8. Kariyone, T. *Saishin shoyakugaku* (Modern Pharmacognosy): 205–207. Tokyo: Hirokawa, 1964.
9. Konno, C. et al. *Planta medica* 35(1979): 150.
10. Kosuga, T. et al. *Yakugaku Zasshi* (Journal of the Pharmaceutical Society of Japan) 98(1978): 1370.
11. Lu, Kuei-sheng. *Chung yo ko hsueh hua ta tzu tien* (Dictionary of the Development of Chinese Medical Science). Hong Kong: n.p., 1954.
12. Miyake, N. *Areruji* (Allergy) 10(1961): 131.
13. Nagoshi, N. and Nakano, K. *Shoyakugaku Zasshi* 30(1976): 42–46.
14. Ninomiya, K. et al. *Journal of Biochemistry* 92(1982): 413.

15. Okano, K. *Kanpo no Rinsho* (Practical Kanpo) 15(1968) nos. 11–12.
16. Pruthi, J. R. *Spices and Condiments: Chemistry, Microbiology, Technology:* Chapter 2. New York: Academic Press, 1980.
17. Saito, Y. *Shoyaku Bunseki Toronkai Koenyoshishu* (Abstracts of the Forum for the Discussion of Pharmacognostic Analysis) 42(1982).
18. Sokai Editorial Department. *Roka o fusegu kanpo no meiyaku* (Popular Kanpo for the Prevention of Aging): 188. Tokyo: Makino, 1978.
19. Tashiro, S. *Kanpo Igaku* (Kanpo Medicine) 9 (1985): 16.
20. Yamauchi, K. and Tsunematsu, T. *Wakan 'Yaku Shinpojumu Kiroku* (Proceedings of the Wakan 'Yaku Symposium) 15(1981/ 82): 29.